M000224176

ORGASM

QUIVER

© 2017 Quarto Publishing Group USA Inc.
Text © 2008, 2010 by Susan Crain Bakos

First Published in 2017 by Fair Winds Press, an imprint of The Quarto Group, 100 Cummings Center, Suite 265-D, Beverly, MA 01915, USA.
T (978) 282-9590 F (978) 283-2742 QuartoKnows.com

Fair Winds Press titles are also available at discount for retail, wholesale, promotional, and bulk purchase. For details, contact the Special Sales Manager by email at specialsales@quarto.com or by mail at The Quarto Group, Attn: Special Sales Manager, 401 Second Avenue North, Suite 310, Minneapolis, MN 55401, USA.

The Publisher maintains the records relating to images in this book required by 18 USC 2257. Records are located at The Quarto Group, 100 Cummings Center, Suite 265-D, Beverly, MA 01915, USA.

The content for this book originally appeared in *The Little Book of the Big Orgasm* (Quiver Books, 2010) and *The Orgasm Bible* (Quiver Books, 2008), both by Susan Crain Bakos.

21 20 19 18 17   1 2 3 4 5

ISBN: 978-1-59233-796-5

Digital edition published in 2017

Library of Congress Cataloging-in-Publication Data available

Cover design/illustration: www.gordonbeveridge.com
Book layout by Sporto

Printed and bound in Hong Kong

Contents

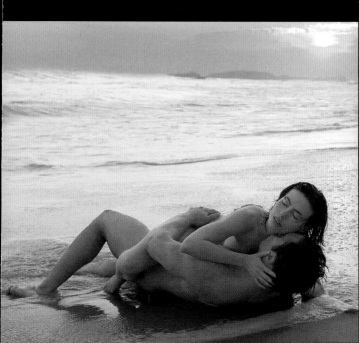

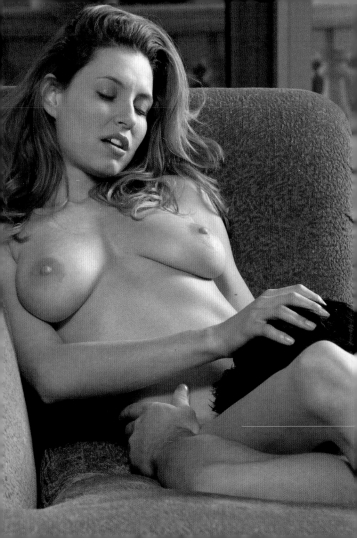

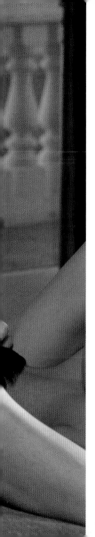

Introduction

This book may be small enough to fit in your handbag, but it's packed with advice for getting, receiving, or having as many orgasms as you want. These 50 fun and sexy games will teach you tips and techniques for achieving your best orgasms yet.

Tap into Two Senses

GAME 1

The Sexy Setup

Text your lover and tell him you need help discovering your special hot spots while you practice your arousal visualization techniques.

Rules & Tools

Select your visual arousal image, such as a red rose, purple orchid, or sunset on a beach. Select a favorite perfume to match your image, or just use a familiar scent. (This isn't the time to try something new. Use a scent that's already known to your lover.) Bring a blindfold or silk ties for gentle bondage if desired.

Playing the Game

Sweet and safe: Before you greet your lover, undress and spray your perfume on any area that you consider a hot spot. Blindfold him and lead him to your bed or a soft rug. Lay down, completely naked, and close your eyes. Practice visualizing your arousal image, but tell him to use only his nose to seek out your hot spots.

Hot and Spicy: Pick a favorite beverage or food that smells and tastes good, such as a dab of dessert wine or after-dinner drink or a smear of chocolate or honey. Blindfold

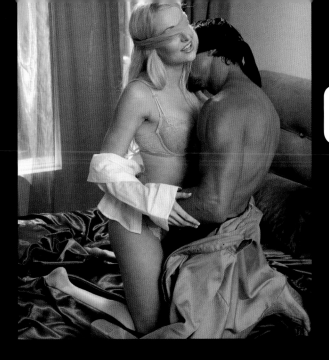

your partner and lead him to your bed or soft rug. Prepare
your body by dabbing the wine, alcohol, chocolate, or honey
on your hot spots, then instruct your lover to lightly tie
your hands above your head. Ask him to lick, smell, nuzzle,
and kiss his way around your body while you practice your
arousal visualization technique. Reward him with tastes
of the actual food or sips of your favorite beverage. If he
comes up hungry for more reapply and replay as needed!

Anatomy Test

The Sexy Setup

It's time for a little hands-on anatomy lesson, and a his-and-her-hot-spot quiz to follow—if you can make it that far!

Rules & Tools

Set up a cozy spot for exploration, such as a soft rug or a freshly made bed. Undress and sit together completely naked. (Alternatively, undress each other slowly with your eyes closed before the next step.) Read the introduction to this book together to learn about all the potential different hot spots. Take notes, make jokes, or come up with sexy names for the various hot spots so you can remember them later on. Bring a blindfold, silk ties for gentle bondage, and edible body paint if desired.

Playing the Game

Sweet and safe: Blindfold your lover and tell him to locate all your various hot spots using only one of the following: his hands, his tongue, his lips, or his fingers. When he's done with his hands, move on one-by-one to his tongue, lips, and fingers. Alternatively, have him blindfold you before he tests his hot-spot knowledge; this allows you to focus completely

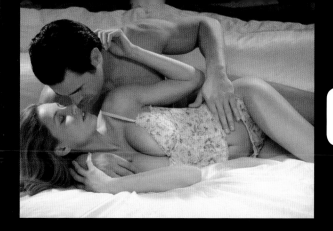

on your arousal visualization image and enjoy every sensation. Switch places.

Hot and Spicy: Before you play the game, use the edible body paint to mark your body with numbers, letters, or other personal symbols, selecting one "marking" per hot spot. Use the order of the markings to indicate which spots are hottest for you, such as #1 for clitoris, #2 for nipples, and so on. Don't forget the less obvious hot spots, such as your lower back, the inside of your wrists, or the base of your throat. Let him blindfold and/or gently restrain you, then call out the numbers or markings to him as he explores your body. For variation, blindfold him and instruct him to visit each mark using his tongue, his finger, or his lips only. Switch places and let him use the paint while you do the exploring!

9

Crisscross Applesauce

(aka Now You've Got the Shivers!)

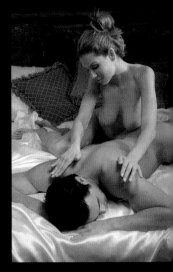

The Sexy Setup

Remember the children's game Crisscross Applesauce? Then you know the goal of this game: to bring out the shivers on your lover's body.

Rules & Tools

All you need is a fingernail, feather, or other small, gentle scratching device for creating the shivers. Set up a sensual spot for exploration and keep some paper and a pen nearby for taking notes. Get naked together in whatever way you desire or come to the game undressed.

Playing the Game

Sweet and safe: Have your lover lay flat on his stomach. Straddle his bottom, sitting on his rear end or lower back. Whisper this rhyme as you make the movements in parentheses:

> Crisscross (draw an X on his back)
> applesauce (rub his back lightly in a circular motion with several fingernails)
> Spiders crawling up your back (walk your fingernails up his back)
> Spiders here (tickle gently under his left arm),
> spiders there (and under his right)
> Spiders even in your hair (lightly tickle his neck, hairline, and head)
> Cool breeze (blow softly at his neckline),
> tight squeeze (squeeze his neck or shoulders)
> Now you've got the shivers! (run your fingernails up and down his back or anywhere close by)

Hot and Spicy: As you draw the X on his back, gently sweep your clitoris and labia across his buttocks. Brush your breasts across his lower back as you walk your fingers up his back. As you blow softly on his neckline, run a finger down his spine, around his buttocks, and back up the crevice; alternatively, whisper "hot air" on his neckline and press your breasts into his back. For variation, use the Crisscross Applesauce game on your lover as he lies on his back and alter the words and movements to discover where he gets the most goose bumps sunny side up. Take notes!

The Art of Seduction

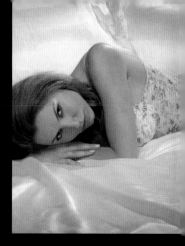

The Sexy Setup

Who says seduction is a lost art? The art of drawn-out flirtation, or sensual interplay between two lovers, can awaken all five of your senses.

Rules & Tools

All you need are a few techniques and someone—your lover or a complete stranger—to practice on. Use your eyes, fingers, and body language to draw your intended victim closer (or create deeper intimacy with a known lover.) This game is best played in an everyday setting; if you set up a sexy scene beforehand, he or she will get wind of what's coming. Instead, make this game a surprise—and the prize is the deep kiss, sizzling foreplay, or extended orgasm that might follow!

Playing the Game

Sweet and safe: Flirting—the foreplay of full-blown seduction—starts with the eyes. Gaze at your lover while he's reading, watching television, or otherwise engaged. Think naughty or seductive thoughts about him until he glances up. As you catch his eye, mischievous thoughts with your eyes...then wink quickly and give a brief smile. (Think subtle) Don't talk unless you have to, and keep your movements and thoughts very simple and sensual. If he glances away, then glances back, play with your hair seductively and let it fall over one eye. Dip your chin slightly but keep your eyes up, then mentally undress him with a penetrating stare. Your eyes will widen slightly at this erotic thought and should, in turn, clue him in to what you're thinking. If he doesn't get the message, move on to the techniques outlined in Hot and Spicy.

Hot and Spicy: Use those cliché flirting moves, such as tossing your hair or crossing and uncrossing your legs, to continue sending subliminal messages to your lover. Toussle your hair (as if you just got finished making love) as you gaze into his eyes. Or slowly run your finger from your throat to your cleavage, mentally transmitting your naughty thoughts. Eat finger foods and slowly lick your fingers or lean forward to expose a quick glimpse of your cleavage. If you stand up to go to the bathroom, turn around and wink at him, then swing your hips ever so slightly as you walk away. If you're sitting next to him, lean close and let your breast touch his upper arm. Use these non verbal clues to tease him into submission—or just draw out the flirtation as long as you like!

Touch Me Here

The Sexy Setup

This game can be played alone or as a couple, but either way it will help heighten the romance and sensuality in your relationship. Text your lover and tell him you've got a touchy feely game that's sure to pique his interest.

Rules & Tools

This game is about investigating the tools that you and your partner find sexy and stimulating. As you discover what you both like, you'll build a set of props and tools to use over and over in your love play. Start by setting a seductive scene, lighting a few candles, and perhaps opening a bottle of wine or champagne. Keep some paper and a pen nearby for taking notes.

Playing the Game

Sweet and safe: Ponder the word "sensual" and what it means to both of you. What do you find sexy or stimulating? Ask your partner what he or she finds sensual. Sexy lingerie? You wearing his shirt (and nothing else)? Him brushing or washing your hair? Create a private list for your eyes only. Take turns practicing (and perfecting) your favorite sensual activities, then set up a weekly or monthly "meeting" to review your list, prioritize your favorites, and experiment with new ideas.

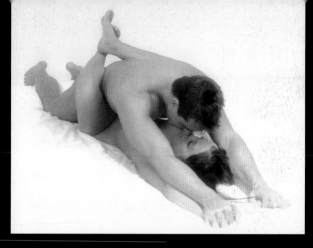

Hot and Spicy: For this version of the game, explore what the word *sensual* means in a tactile way: Play with the fabrics you find the most *sensual* on bare skin. Pull out your softest cashmere sweater or wrap, silk scarves or gloves, fur accessories, a feather, any other clothing or fabric, then use them to touch and caress each other's bodies. Slowly sweep the silk across his throat, tease his nipples with a caress of velvet, tickle his lower back with a feather, or stroke his penis with a cashmere-covered hand. As you play, don't forget to brush your nipples across his lips, run a finger around his genitals, or lightly kiss his lower back and buttocks. Eventually your travels can lead you to massaging each other with velvet-, fur-, or cashmere-covered hands, stimulating her clitoris with the hint of a silk scarf, or tickling each other's lips, throat, or nipples with a feather. Remember, the better the fabric or object feels on bare skin, the higher the "sizzle" factor.

Flex Test

The Sexy Setup

Text or email your lover and tell him you need to work out—but it's your PC muscles that need exercise, and you need him as your personal trainer.

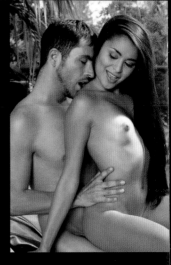

Rules & Tools

You can play this game with your own finger, your lover's finger, a vibrator, a set of Kegel exercisers, such as Candida Royalle's little barbell, or your lover's penis. Bring lubrication if needed (make sure you're relaxed and/or lubricated before playing).

Playing the Game

Sweet and safe: Get naked together in whatever way suits your mood—alone or with each other. Be sure you're in a frame of mind (and location) where you can concentrate, as this exercise takes some focus. Ask your partner to help you get excited, but don't go too far—you want to be wet (naturally or with lubrication) but not begging for release.

Then settle back in a comfortable place, close your eyes, and practice using your PC muscles while your partner watches—or assists. Start with your partner's finger: Practice pulling his finger into your vagina using your PC muscles, then expel it the same way. Pull in, then push out. When you've mastered that move, try it with the little barbell. In and out, in and out. If this is your first time, don't overwork your muscles—hand the reins over to your partner and let him take over from there! Alternatively, practice on any of the toys, but let him kiss your nipples or finger your clitoris at the same time for a double-barreled sensation.

Hot and Spicy: Practice the same moves, but this time use your lover's erect penis or a vibrator. Try quick, rhythmic pulses....then long, slow squeezing. If this move is new to you, try sitting astride your lover and closing your eyes so you can really focus. While it might be hard to tune out all the pleasurable sensations you're feeling, do your best to concentrate on the one move— and ask your lover if he can feel the sensation of your muscles gripping and releasing! Mix up your timing and rhythm depending on what feels good. If he comes close to orgasm, pull away to draw out the sensation and prolong the pleasure.

Bring Out the Big Cats

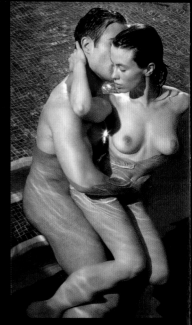

The Sexy Setup

You know you're a tiger in the jungle, and your lover is a lion—better known as King of the Plains. Now use this role-play game to see who rules the bedroom!

Rules & Tools

All you need is yourself, but adding tiger stripes using body paint, wearing tiger-striped lingerie, or messing up your hair and purring softly can heighten the effects! Be sure to ask your lover to play the part of a lion, otherwise known as a big cat who wants to be in charge.

Playing the Game

Sweet and safe: Play like a lusty tigress while your lover watches. Get down on all fours, then lean forward (show off your cleavage!) with your weight on your arms and your butt in the air. Rock your pelvis from side to side, then slowly crawl across the room like a cat in heat. As you crawl closer to your lover, lower your head and slowly lick his toes, ankles, or lower legs. As you travel upward on his body, practice squeezing and releasing your PC muscles and inhaling and exhaling in time. Lick, nibble, and gently bite your way around your lover's body, then reverse roles and let him play the stalking lion. You can be submissive—or battle it out for bedroom domination!

Hot and Spicy: Pretend you're a stalking, hungry tigress that's spotted her next meal. Get down on all fours, then lean forward with your breasts near the floor and your butt in the air. Start a vigorous back-and-forth rocking motion with your pelvis and give a gentle growl from your throat. Spot your prey—your lover's penis, his mouth, or his nipples and lean forward, inhale, and gently squeeze your buttocks together. Then push your body back, putting more weight on your knees than on your arms. As you exhale, relax your pelvis and buttocks. Repeat the movements as needed as you move in for the kill!

Playing with Kundalini Fire

The Sexy Setup

Text or email your lover and tell her you want to practice some sexual yoga moves together. If she hesitates, remind her that lovers who practice yoga together often come together!

Rules & Tools

Find a large, open space—such as a living room rug or a large blanket in the woods—for your sexual yoga. Wear loose (or little) clothing, and bring along plenty of focus (and a dash of sexual tension!).

Playing the Game

Sweet and safe: Connecting Energies: Facing each other with knees bent, make eye contact and breathe together, inhaling and exhaling in time. Open up your arms and hold them around your lover, first without touching. Then hold your partner loosely by the shoulders and breathe together for a few minutes. Feel the sexual energy pulsating through your body and into hers. Practice this technique while you gently run your fingers up and down her arms, around her lower back, and under her bottom. See how long you can

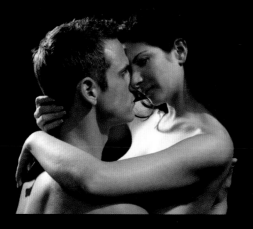

resist kissing each other while you practice breathing, touching, and sharing energy. Reward each other with a long passionate kiss, then try the advanced moves.

Hot and Spicy: Rising Energies: Face each other at arm's length apart and hold hands. Bounce gently together. Then slowly squat down to the floor. Resting on the balls of your feet, rock gently, supporting each other through your clasped hands. Feel the Kundalini energy uncoiling inside your bodies. Now slowly rise together. As you rise, the Kundalini rises inside each of you. Repeat the squatting and rising, moving rhythmically. After a few times, focus on coordinating your breathing together. Repeat several times, then transfer the energy to your lips for gentle kisses, your hands for lusty caresses, or your genitals for rhythmic pulsing.

Kissing 101

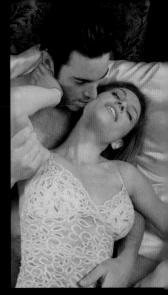

The Sexy Setup

No matter how long you've been with your current lover or partner, it's never too late to revisit the basics of kissing. Think back to the days when you first met your partner and how you learned what kind of kisses he or she liked, then tell him or her you'd like a refresher course to reignite your intimacy and passion.

Rules & Tools

All you really need for this game is an open mind, a set of healthy lips, and a sense of adventure, but bring along flavored lip glosses, a silk scarf for gentle bondage, or your favorite sex toys for variety.

Playing the Game

Sweet and safe: Pretend that you're meeting your lover for the first time. You've never kissed before, but you know you want each other. Study the shape of his or her lips, noticing if they're thin or full or red or rosy. Outline the shape of her lips with your finger, tracing around her mouth and perhaps stroking her cheek. Ask her what she likes best (or what she likes least) when it comes to liplock. As she describes what she likes, listen, then try to demonstrate like a student following his master. Ask her, "Like this?" Tell her, "Show me." The more you listen—and try to respond in kind—the more she's likely to open up to you, and we all know where that can lead. Ready for more advanced kissing? Lean toward her and use the tip of your tongue to ever so gently tickle her lips, or brush your lips across her lips in a slow and sensual movement. If she's willing, very gently nibble or suck her lower lip, explore the tip of her tongue, or lick her lips.

Hot and Spicy: Ready for Kissing 201? Try these techniques. If you'd like her to relax and open her mouth, gently probe with the tip of your tongue. Alternatively, if your partner offers too much tongue, whisper "let's try using just the very tippy top of our tongues" or some other soft and gentle means of redirecting the kissing play. When you're ready, practice (or reinvent) the art of French kissing. Alternatively, have her apply flavored lip gloss so you can guess the flavor—and explore new sensations! Next up: Back her against a wall, hold her hands above her head, and explore her mouth, neck, and cleavage with your lips, tongue, and mouth. And last but not least, come back to the kiss—deep or gentle, light or hard—that makes her melt inside.

Bump and Grind

The Sexy Setup

Take a trip back in time for this game: Back to the days when making out was considered "fast" and "going all the way" was something you might save for marriage.

Rules & Tools

All you need for this game is a healthy dose of restraint—and I don't mean bondage! You may want to select your attire depending on how you want the game to go: Lightweight tops and short skirts on her, for example, may make it easier to simulate intercourse fully clothed!

Playing the Game

Sweet and safe: Set the rules from the start: This version of the game has to take place fully clothed. You can kiss, fondle, caress, grope, grab, and stimulate each other in any way you desire, but it all has to take place without removing any clothing—and standing up. When you feel the steam rising between the two of you, bump against him on the upstroke and grind into him on the downstroke. Wrap one leg around his waist or use a door or wall for balance—but don't lie down. The goal? To orgasm without actually touching bare skin. Then make a modern game of cleaning up—jump in the shower together or take a long, hot bath.

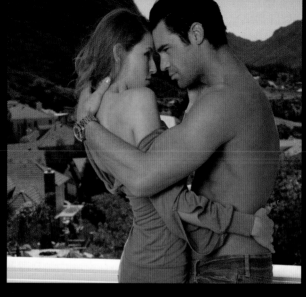

Hot and Spicy: Remember when you were a teenager and you made out on the family room floor while your parents were sleeping upstairs? You kept your clothes on—the better for a quick recovery if the parents came in. And it was really hot. This "outercourse" or "dry humping" game is similar to bump and grind, but you simulate any intercourse position you want, whether it's him on top in bed, her on top on the sofa, or grind from behind on the floor! See if you can stop before you reach orgasm, or don't hold back—let the juices flow! Jump in the shower (and throw those clothes in the laundry!) when the game is over.

Think Yourself Off

The Sexy Setup

Some women can have an orgasm just by having their nipples sucked or their inner thighs kissed, and nothing else. An even smaller number of luckier ones can reach orgasm via fantasy alone. This game lets you try your hand at the ultimate mind-body-fantasy connection!

Rules & Tools

Establish an erotic mood with candles, wine, sexy clothing, or music—whatever turns you on. You can play the sweet and safe version of this game while you're alone, then graduate to the hot and spicy version with your lover. The sweet and safe version can also be used for arousal prior to your lover's arrival—especially if you're having a quickie!

Playing the Game

Sweet and safe: Create a lush, passionate fantasy—and make it graphic. Take a dozen deep breaths, then a dozen shallow ones. Use your breath to create and foster your own physical desire. Flex your PC muscles in time with your panting. As you breath and flex, let your mind relax, having your fantasy help build the sexual desire. If you can't reach orgasm by thought alone, slowly introduce other elements,

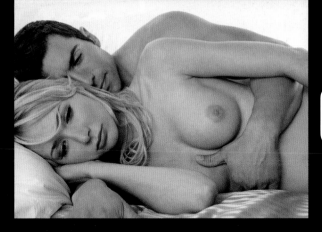

such as caressing your belly, squeezing your nipples, or palming your "sex mound." Try to hold off from masturbating with your hand or vibrator unless you absolutely have to, and remember that getting even halfway to orgasm is a great start.

Hot and Spicy: Invite your partner or lover to come along for the ride. You set the ground rules: He or she can watch but not touch; touch in certain instances or places; or jump fully into the game upon your command. Communicate your favorite fantasy. Take a dozen deep breaths, then a dozen shallow ones. Use your breath and visualization to create physical desire. Describe what you're imagining in detail to your lover. If it turns you on, have him respond or add his own details. If you can't think yourself off this way, invite your partner to join in at any point to help you orgasm.

Couple Fantasy Encounters

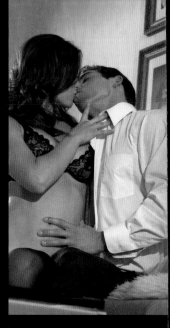

The Sexy Setup

Tell your lover that the couple that fantasizes together often comes together—and you've got a special game for doing just that. Ask him to start imagining a fantasy the two of you can act out but to be prepared for using more than just his imagination!

Rules & Tools

This game is simple in concept: Create a fantasy and write its script together, then act it out over a one-week time frame. Depending on your fantasy, you may need to assemble or purchase various props. Make a list once you've progressed to the appropriate stage. On the day of the "encounter" be sure to set a private, sensual scene where your couple fantasy can come to life!

Playing the Game

Sweet and safe: On the first night, talk about fantasy scenarios and select one that you both find arousing. The key is choosing a fantasy that will arouse both of you.) On days two through six, email one another with ideas for the plot, and then take a little time each night before you go to bed to write your script together. If it makes you hot, all the better! (You may want to hold off on having sex during the scripting stage in order to build sexual tension.) Write erotic and descriptive dialogue, such as "The curve of your hips in the candlelight was like a sensuous sliver of the moon in the sky." Don't be afraid to go over the top. Assemble props—masks, costumes, sex toys—ahead of time, or think about playing with edible body paints, food, or other edible props. On the last day, act out your script together as if you were presenting an erotic play—and be prepared for mind-blowing orgasms!

Hot and Spicy: Imagine you're creating a magazine article about your fantasy encounter and take photos along the way; envision a storyboard of your fantasy with notes, the script, photos, and props as your building blocks. Alternatively, try filming your actions during the week, culminating with filming your erotic fantasy as you act it out. Ready for even more action? Invite an audience to watch (but not participate). If you're really ready to step it up, create and act out a fantasy that includes another woman, another man, or even another couple.

The Queen of Orgasm

The Sexy Setup

Many women fantasize about being dominant, in part because usually it's the male who takes the lead. Here's a game with many different flavors and variations that allows the woman to command the troops!

Rules & Tools

There's only one rule in this game: what you say goes. The tools will vary depending on your fantasy: If you're the queen and

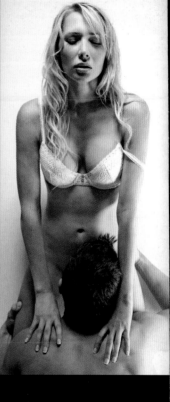

he's your prince, then pull out an old bridesmaid's dress and act the part. If you're the mistress and he's the sex slave, then pull out those black boots, don a leather jacket, and borrow a riding crop for gentle sex play.

Playing the Game

Sweet and safe: Tell your lover the theme for your domination game, then dress (or undress!) appropriately. You're the boss, and his job is to service you—in whatever way turns you on (and gets you off!) the most. Want him to get on his knees and eat you out? Tell him. Wishing he'd lather your whole body in lotion and massage you to orgasm? Say the word. Want him to watch you masturbate while he films it? Issue your orders!

Hot and Spicy: Here's where you can step it up, either by introducing props or letting out your dominant, dirty, or naughty side. When you're wearing boots and leather, use the riding crop for a few gentle taps on his naked behind. If you really like the idea of a sex slave, keep him naked for several hours on a Sunday afternoon—and at your beck and call, whether it's for sex, food, or laundry! Alternatively, have your way with him—try tying his hands to the bedposts, then ride him like a cowgirl. Don't let him loose until he's come three times, even if he begs for release. Or tie his hands up and tease him, whether that means stimulating him or yourself (or both)! Whatever gets you (or him) off, make it happen—but remember you're the boss.

Handyman Cum Calling

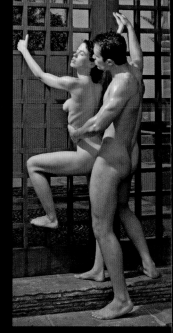

The Sexy Setup

This is every stay-at-home mom's fantasy: the hot and randy handyman who's handy in more ways than one! Tell your lover you've got a secret game for her, but you're not going to tell her what it is until the game begins. She doesn't need to do anything special—except be home alone when you come knocking!

Rules & Tools

Dress the part—put on a pair of dirty jeans, work boots, and a big sweatshirt or heavy jacket. Borrow a tool belt and load it up with sex toys, lubricant, or silk ties, but keep it under your jacket or in a bucket or shopping bag so she doesn't see it at first.

Playing the Game

Sweet and safe: Ring the doorbell. When she answers, tell her you're the handyman whose come to help around the house. Ask her what needs fixing. Are her drawers squeaky? Do the bedsprings need attention? Depending on her answer, lead her to the room where you can best play the game, then tell her you're handy in more ways than one. Ask her where your hands are most needed: To undress her slowly? To caress her breasts and nipples? To stimulate her clitoris? Then get to work!

Hot and Spicy: Ring the doorbell, introduce yourself, and take charge. Lead her from room to room, slowly building the seduction and asking her what she needs fixed. Offer to change the lightbulb, but brush up against her suggestively, kiss her ankles as you pretend to look under the couch, or grab her from behind as she moves from room to room. Once you've settled on a room, take off your coat and show her your tools, then tell her you're especially handy with tools that penetrate, applying lubricant where it's most needed, and screwing things in. Demonstrate just how handy you are until she's hot and wet, then strip down and nail her on the floor. Ready to take it up a notch? Surprise your lover by wearing a tool belt—and nothing else. Make yourself hard before you walk in the room and she's sure to melt at the sight of her favorite tool!

Back to School

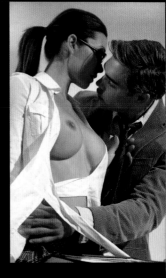

The Sexy Setup

Ask your lover if he's ready to return to the schoolhouse, but this time his courses will include some hot and naughty fantasy play! Then get ready to dress up like a schoolgirl or the hot and sexy teacher who he's always fantasized about.

Rules & Tools

Dress the part of a schoolgirl: short blue skirt, white blouse, and white knee-highs. If you're feeling really daring, skip the underwear. To play the part of a teacher, try a low-cut white blouse, thigh-high white garters, a skirt, and high heels! Set up the scene beforehand—have a ruler, pencils, notebooks, and a desk ready for your game, and stash lubricant, sex toys, and silk ties in the drawers.

Playing the Game

Sweet and safe (schoolgirl): Invite your lover into the schoolhouse and lead him to his seat, perhaps flashing a glimpse of your upper thigh or bare bottom. Talk him through an overview of your course notes, all the while flouncing your skirt, bending over suggestively, or playing with your hair. Ready to tease him further? Sit on his lap and play with his hair, then put his hand on your thigh and tell him today's lesson is anatomy. To step it up a notch, grab his package, kiss and then pull away, or play with yourself while he watches—then tell him you've been naughty and you need a good spanking!

Hot and spicy (teacher): Pick a lesson for the day— anatomy, biology, even sexual response—and talk about the course as you walk around the room, all the while flashing your leg, leaning over his desk to show your cleavage, or slapping the ruler gently on your hand. As you quiz him on his knowledge, slowly remove your skirt or blouse, all the while staring directly into his eyes. Reward him with a kiss or a touch of your breast if he answers a question correctly, but then move away so the teasing tension continues to build. Continue removing your clothing, then kiss the back of his neck as you stroke his chest from behind, or order him to kiss your breasts, fondle your bottom, stroke your thighs, or even lick your clitoris—but always pull away at some point to continue teasing. Ready for the final exam? Position yourself on the desk and invite him over! Alternatively, surprise him by reversing roles: Get into a gentle struggle (but let him win). Have him tie you to the chair or desk, then either tease you into submission or take you while you fight back.

Mutual Masturbation

The Sexy Setup

If you're looking for a little fun and relaxation (and perhaps a break from pleasuring each other), this is the game for you. Tell your partner you're going to share the pleasure tonight, but each one of you controls your own destiny!

Rules & Tools

Create a seduction scene exactly as you would do for "having sex": Dim the lights or light some candles and put on some music. Arrange piles of pillows both for comfort and good positions for watching each other get off.

Playing the Game

Sweet and safe: Feeling a little shy? Start by having a glass of wine. Don't strip naked. Instead, don an open shirt worn alone or thigh-highs, heels, and a bustier. Start by flirting your way into it, as if you and your partner were getting ready to be together. Then slowly move away and relax into the process. Close your eyes if you need to, then run your hands over your body the way you like to be touched. Fondle or squeeze your nipples, caress your thighs, and run your fingers lightly over your clitoris. Apply lubricant if needed and slowly circle your pubic mound, teasing the clitoris.

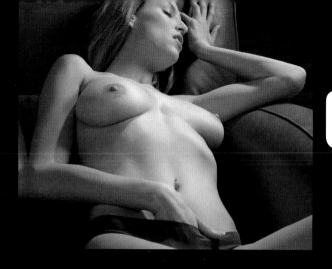

Draw it out like this, pretending you're alone if you feel at all self-conscious. Chances are he's touching himself, too.

Hot and Spicy: Take turns masturbating—but stopping just before orgasm—then let your partner do the same. This kind of starting and stopping, all the while watching each other, can really prolong the pleasure—and heighten the orgasm. Alternatively, ask your partner to play a partial role, such as fondling your nipples from behind while you caress your clitoris. (Don't be surprised if he tries to slip his penis inside you once you've come!) If he likes it, stroke his nipples while he masturbates, nibble on his neck, lightly caress his lower back, or lick your way up his thighs. The combination of his own touch and your involvement is sure to send him over the edge.

Masturbation Slave

The Sexy Setup

Tell your lover that you've got a game he's sure to love (especially if he likes being dominated). Tell him you're the beautiful Middle-Eastern princess, and he's the handsome masturbation slave who has to touch himself whenever his mistress desires.

Rules & Tools

Dress in your favorite Middle-Eastern princess outfit: Put on your sexiest bikini-style top, bikini bottoms, sheer skirt and a decorative belt, choker, and arm bands. Dress your lover in a loincloth or nothing at all. Assemble a pair of handcuffs, choker, or other props as desired.

Playing the Game

Sweet and safe: Order your lover to touch himself while you watch. If you want him to caress your breasts, suck your nipples, or squeeze your buttocks at the same time, order him to do so until you want him to stop. Don't let him orgasm—order him to stop from time to time, then mix in

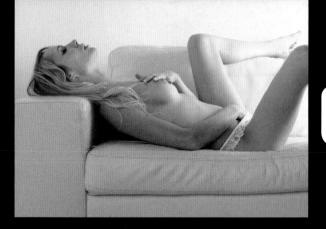

having him hand-feed you, massage your shoulders, or even watch a sexy movie together. Make him and start and stop masturbating at your whim—and tease him by masturbating yourself.

Hot and Spicy: Buy your lover a choker and leash and lead him from room to room like a dog. When you want him to masturbate, tell him to do it (or face punishment). Keep a paddle or crop on hand for gently punishing his failure to use proper enthusiasm or for showing any sign of disrespect. Ready to really step it up a notch? Make your lover masturbate in a public place, such as a parked car or a spot in the woods, while you watch! Remember, you're in charge!

Learn His Strokes

The Sexy Setup

Most men masturbate in the same direct way, but this game involves you learning a variety of different strokes and testing which ones he likes best. Tell your lover you're ready for a "knowledge transfer" between his masturbatory hand and your hands, fingers, and palms.

Rules & Tools

Set a sexy scene, whether that means putting clean, silky sheets on the bed, setting up a soft rug in front of the fireplace, or lighting candles in your bathroom and getting into the tub together!

Playing the Game

Sweet and safe: Ask him to demonstrate each of the following techniques, then try to replicate the stroke yourself. Slowly caress the base of his penis, squeezing the shaft and massaging the base. Take his penis in one hand and stroke slowly up and down the shaft with your thumb or fingers from the other hand. Vary the pressure. Circle the head of his penis with the flat of your hand, using any tiny drops of semen as lubrication while you rub your palm around. Use both hands on the shaft and perform the up-and-down stroke in slow motion.

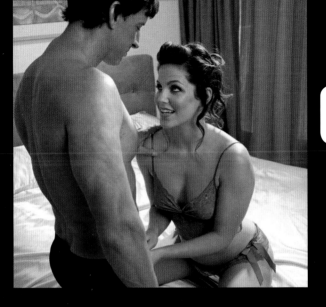

Hot and Spicy: Ready to take it up a notch? Put the flat of one hand over the head of his penis. Use the fingers of the other hand to stroke the shaft. Vary the pressure and speed—and ask him for verbal feedback. At the end of an up-down stroke, lightly squeeze the head of his penis while you kiss him deeply. Last but not least, lay his penis in the palm of your hand and close your fingertips lightly around it, using a slow, light stroke while keeping the hand open. This feels more like a caress than a stroke, and it slows him down. It's the male stroking version of "taking the time to smell the roses."

Door-to-Door Vibrator Salesman

The Sexy Setup

This fantasy game is purrrrrfect for men who like to role-play...and pull out all the toys! Just dress in a suit and pretend to be a door-to-door vibrator salesman. Try and surprise your lover when she thinks you're off at work or busy doing something else.

Rules & Tools

You'll need a suit, briefcase, pamphlets, and most important of all, a selection of vibrators.

Playing the Game

Sweet and safe: Ring the doorbell, then come into the house and explain that you have some very exciting products to show her. Take out the vibrators one by one, taking your time handling each one and explaining which are best suited for what types of play. Ask her if she'd like to borrow one and try it out (with you watching, of course)!

Hot and Spicy: Come into the house and lay down the rules: You can only show her the products if she's naked, so the first thing she has to do is strip down (or get into

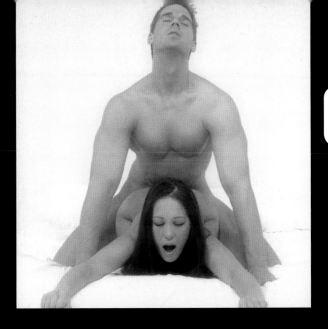

something comfortable, like a short and sexy bathrobe). What's more, you're going to demonstrate their effectiveness on her, whether she likes it or not. At this point you can pull out some silk ties or handcuffs and bind her arms or legs to a chair leg. Then run through the product line one by one, taking as much time as you like to demonstrate just how effective the devices are for stimulation, teasing, and perhaps even orgasm. Ready to step it up a notch? Ask her swap roles and test the vibrators on you—perhaps you'd like to try anal stimulation!

Finger Fun

The Sexy Setup

Call your lover and tell her you've got some fingers that are itching to do some exploring and some toys that will add to the fun. Remember to use her fingers as well as yours!

Rules & Tools

You'll need an assortment of finger toys for this game or a selection of miniature vibrators.

Playing the Game

Sweet and safe: Kiss your lover passionately, nuzzle her neck, and slowly undress her with both hands. Have her lie down or get comfortable in a sofa chair, then start at her toes. Arming yourself with your finger toys or miniature vibrators, tickle her every fantasy. Lick her toes while you finger her labia, then move up to nibble her thighs while she stimulates her clitoris. Have her squeeze her own nipples while you add some tongue action, then move back to her masturbating and you using the finger toy on her nipples. She's sure to experience a mind-blowing orgasm!

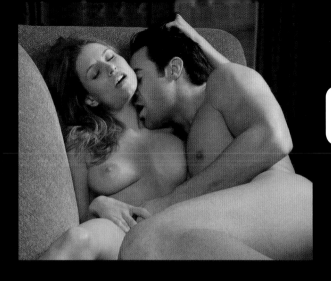

Hot and Spicy: Get your lover hot and wet, then ask her to kneel on all fours so you can enter her from behind. As you slowly penetrate her from behind, have her stimulate her clitoris using the finger vibrator. Try to time your climaxes together. Alternatively, have her use the finger vibrator on your nipples, perineum, or other hot spots while you masturbate to orgasm.

Queen of Foreplay

(Hands-on Foreplay for Her)

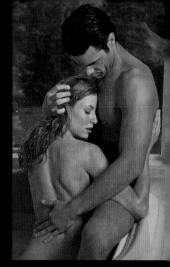

The Sexy Setup

Here's a game where she gets to be queen—and you're the prince who's come to charm her with your spectacular foreplay techniques.

Rules & Tools

Set a sensual scene for your encounter. Leave the sex toys in the drawer for tonight and focus on using just your own mouth and hands to drive her crazy with desire.

Playing the Game

Sweet and safe: Take her face in your hands, kiss her eyelids, and, with one hand still holding her face, stroke her cheeks and forehead with your thumb. As you kiss her mouth or neck, massage her breasts with the flat of your hand, then slip off her blouse and bra in a slow, sensual movement. Once her breasts are bare, glide your hand, with the first two fingers open in a V, up each of her breasts, catching her nipple in the V. Now kiss that nipple. Take her nipple gently between two fingers and pinch. Slip off her remaining clothes, caress her inner thighs from her knees up. Let your thumb or fingers graze her vulva as you reach the top of her thighs. Don't forget to caress her back, shoulders, legs and belly. Is she moaning with desire?

Hot and Spicy: Use light circular motions with your fingertips on her genital area. Part her labia and make long strokes on the outside lips. Then curve one or two fingers and use the space between the knuckle and joint to massage her inner and outer lips lightly in a back-and-forth motion. Alternate that stroke with one using your thumb or first finger alone. Rotate your fingers around her clitoris, alternating a clockwise and counterclockwise motion. Stroke down with one finger on either side of her clitoris, rotate, and stroke down again. If she likes direct clitoral stimulation, take the clitoris between two fingers and gently rotate. But if, like many women, she can't stand the intensity of that stroke, circle your fingertips above the clitoris (at the twelve o'clock point). Ready for more? Add the G-spot stroke. While continuing the twelve o'clock rotation on her clitoris, insert a finger or two into her vagina and massage her G-spot. Continue to stroke her clitoris as you massage her G-spot, and don't be surprised if she ejaculates during this mind-blowing orgasm.

King of Foreplay

(Hands-on Foreplay for Him)

The Sexy Setup

Here's a chance to pay back your lover for all the wonderful things he's done for you. Text him that your dying to practice some newfound foreplay techniques. Chances are just the message will get him hard!

Rules & Tools

Create a lusty lair with soft blankets, animal rugs, or other sensual fabrics. Put on some soft music, light a few candles, and open a bottle of wine. If desired, use your imagination and dress like a subject in King Henry the Eighth's lusty court: Cleavage is a must, and perhaps a long skirt with no underwear underneath!

Playing the Game

Sweet and safe: Knead his shoulders and back very gently to help him relax. Make circular motions with your hands on his back from the spine upward and to the sides of his body. Alternate the circular motions with smooth, gliding strokes. Remove his shirt as you kiss the nape of his neck, then slowly remove his pants and underwear. Try single-or two-finger gliding strokes on his inner thighs, back, and the sides of his neck, then repeat the long, gliding strokes on his chest, stomach, and thighs. Do something entirely unexpected: Use the single-finger stroke on his face and the delicate areas around his eyelids and ears. Run your finger along his throat as you kiss him deep and hard to along the base of his neck and down his chest.

Hot and Spicy: Kneel between his legs, occasionally kissing or stroking his inner thighs. Take his testicles one at a time very gently between your fingers and thumb, then hold a testicle in the palm of your hand and tickle it lightly with the pads of your fingers. If he likes it, repeat on the other side. If he's not comfortable, move on to his golden shaft. Hold the base of his penis in one hand and work your other hand in a circular, upwardly twisting movement to the head. Use the palm of that hand to caress the head of his penis. Take his penis in both hands. Imagine building a fire with his penis as the stick: Using a rolling/rubbing motion, starting at the base. Roll/rub up to the head, keeping his penis between your palms. Use only upward motions. Start over at the base when you reach the head. Start slowly. Increase the speed as he gets closer to orgasm. Lean forward so that he ejaculates onto your breasts!

Reviving a Fallen Soldier

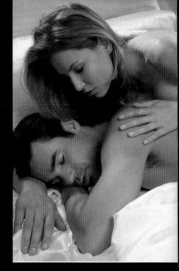

The Sexy Setup

Every man, at some time or another, has lost his erection. No worries—just use one of the techniques outlined to turn his game back on!

Rules & Tools

Rule number one: Don't make a big deal of it, and don't take it personally. Instead, go with the flow—and remind him how you love being with him, regardless of whether his solider is ready for battle!

Playing the Game

Sweet and safe: Ask him to focus on you for awhile. Have him kiss, caress, stroke, and fondle you—or even give you orgasm using his tongue. Chances are he'll have an erection after that, but if not, move on to to the Cowgirl in Charge. First, straddle him. Grasp the base of his penis firmly in one hand. Use the head of his penis to stroke your vulva and clitoris. When you are ready, lower yourself onto his penis without letting go of the base. Grasp the first third of his penis in your strong PC muscle. Simulate thrusting with that muscle. (This alone may revive his erection.) Lean forward, supporting yourself on one hand resting beside his body. (Your other hand still has that penis. Don't let go of it.) Work his penis up and down with your hand and PC muscle. Alternate that with "thrusting of the head" stroke, or using the head of his penis against your clitoris.

Hot and Spicy: Sometimes even a good blow job or your best hand job may not be enough to revive a fallen solider. The Stand Up Kiss, works by combining the two. Start by holding his penis firmly in one hand. Take it into your mouth, moving the top third of the shaft in and out. Use the fingers of your other hand to stroke his perineum in a light, ticking fashion. If he responds to gentle scratching, do that. When he becomes erect, use one hand to do a circular twisting motion up the shaft. Then start at the bottom again. At the same time you're twisting up, swirl your tongue around the corona. Alternate the swirl with the butterfly flick— flicking your tongue rapidly across the corona. Continue the hand move while taking his testicles into your mouth, one at a time, and sucking lightly. Flick your tongue rapidly across his perineum. Go back to the head of his penis and alternate swirling, flicking, and sucking. Remember: Don't take his penis too far into your mouth when you suck or you won't be able to pull off the suction.

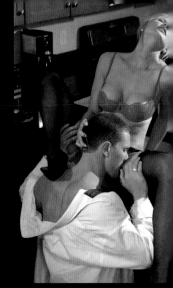

Preheat the Oven

The Sexy Setup

Put away the pots and pans—you'll want to play this racy game of foreplay right on the kitchen counter! Tell your lover that your oven needs preheating. What's more, your drawers are open and you're serving something hot and spicy for dinner.

Rules & Tools

Clean off the counters and dim the lights. Wear an apron with nothing under it and line up some sexy kitchen tools or gadgets, such as a soft pastry brush or a pair of tongs (if you like it a little rougher). Set the timer to however long you want the foreplay to last.

Playing the Game

Sweet and safe: Position yourself on the counter, then ask him to remove your apron using his teeth. Once you're naked, ask him to prepare you for higher temperatures by rubbing you down with massage oil. Make sure he spends ample time on your breasts, rump, and inner thighs. Ready to step it up a notch? Ask your lover to blindfold you with a kitchen towel and turn you on using his choice of kitchen utensils. Have him tickle your inner thighs or genitals with a soft pastry brush, gently pinch your nipples with tongs, blow cool air on your neckline using a turkey baster, and so forth.

Hot and Spicy: Lie on the counter, let your lover blindfold you with a kitchen towel, and ask him to bring out the tray of ice cubes. Start by passing an ice cube back and forth between you while you kiss. Have him hold the cube in his mouth while he explores your body, alternating between an icy tongue and hot breath. The goal: Melt all the ice cubes in the tray. Alternatively, have him lie on the counter and play "heat and ice." While performing fellatio, vary the temperature of your mouth. Start with normal body temperature. Then, using your hand to stimulate his penis, fill your mouth with ice cubes. Wait until your tongue is numb before spitting out the ice. Apply your frozen tongue to his penis. This feels like a jolt of sexual electricity. After a few minutes, when you oral temperature is back to normal, repeat the procedure, this time filling your mouth with a hot liquid. His orgasm is more intense after playing with heat and ice!

Variations on a Theme: Public Foreplay

The Sexy Setup

You've seen that couple who can't keep their hands off each other in a restaurant, at a party, anywhere in public. Maybe you've been that couple. This game is all about trying on different flavors of foreplay, but all of them should take place in public!

Rules & Tools

There's really only one rule here: Don't let your foreplay get out of hand! The goal is to build the tension—and save the release for later, perhaps at home or at the hotel. If you absolutely can't control your passion and you find yourself needing to come in public, just remember not to get caught—being naked in public can be against the law. (On the flip side, the thrill of playing but not getting caught may make your public foreplay even hotter!)

Playing the Game

Sweet and safe: Pick a dark booth in your neighborhood bar. Kick off your shoe and play with his leg—all the way up his leg. Alternatively, sit on his lap on a park bench and make out, or kiss and fondle one another on the beach at

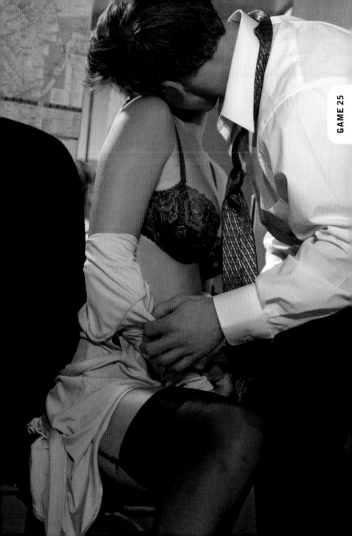

night. Ready to step it up a notch? Consider car sex! You don't have to park on a lover's lane, either—the driveway or garage will do. Part of the thrill in this game is the limited range of motion. The space is tight—and that feels illicit—so try these moves on for size: Push the frontseats as far forward as they go, ask him to lie down on the backseat, and ride him like a cowgirl (with your clothes on!). Have your lover kneel with one leg on each front seat and push his penis toward you over the armrest. You sit in the backseat and suck him (but don't let him come!). Last but not least, get out of the car, sit on the hood, and have him explore your clitoris with his tongue!

Hot and Spicy: Try a game of "ride and tease" on the elevator at work, in a department store, or at the airport. The goal? Tease each other between floors so that once you get home (or back to his office), you can have hot and steamy intercourse. Start the game by getting on the elevator together, push the button for every single floor, and stand at the back. If no one else gets on, kiss, fondle, and touch each other as much as possible before the elevator stops at the next floor and the doors open. If other people are in front of you, discreetly fondle his crotch or let him grab your behind until you're alone again. As the doors open and close, continue this teasing action to build the excitement. Once you reach the top floor, repeat the game on the way down. Better yet, find a hidden stairwell, put one leg up on the railing, and let him enter you standing up to release the pent-up tension!

Pick a Card, Any Card

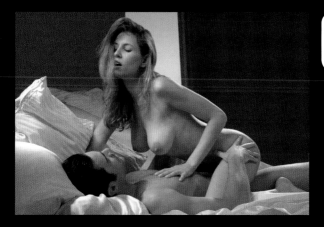

The Sexy Setup

Tell your lover you've got a game of cards that's sure to leave her satisfied. Designate a playing card for each type of female orgasm, then let her pick one for your sex play. If she's been really good let her pick two cards!

Rules & Tools

You'll need between three and six cards, depending on what game you're playing; consider using the aces and queens, for example, or the ace, two, and three of a certain suit.

Create a "cheat sheet" to remember that the ace of hearts represents a clitoral orgasm, the ace of diamonds a vaginal orgasm, the ace of spades a G-spot orgasm, and so on.

Playing the Game

Sweet and safe: Set up a romantic or sensual space for your sex play, whether that's in your bedroom or on a soft rug. This version of the game uses the three cards to represent the "tamest" types of orgasm: clitoral, vaginal, and G-spot. Have your lover pick a card, then focus on giving her that type of orgasm. Alternatively, let her have all three cards, but give her the choice of what order she wants her orgasms in. Or give her multiple versions of the same card.

Hot and Spicy: This version of the game is a little more adventurous! Designate additional cards to represent an anal orgasm, an extra-genital orgasm, and a combination of orgasms. If she picks the anal card, plan on spending a lot of time licking her anus and/or inserting your well-lubed fingers and gently massaging. Working on an extra-genital orgasm? She's more likely to have this type after she's experienced a clitoral orgasm, so throw in a freebee and then turn all your attention to fondling, sucking, licking, pinching, or massaging her nipples, breasts, inner thighs, lower back, or other very sensitive areas. If she picks the combination orgasm card, ask which she prefers: Clitoris and vagina together? Clitoris and anal play? G-spot intercourse and anal play? Any way you cut it, she's sure to hit the jackpot!

Connect the Dots

The Sexy Setup

No surprise here: You can heighten your sex play and orgasms by hitting each other's hot spots during oral and manual stimulation. Why not play a game of mutual hot spot exploration?

Rules & Tools

The sky's the limit with this game—bring along your vibrator, a cock ring for him, or some silk ties for light bondage.

Playing the Game

Hot and spicy (for her): During manual foreplay, stroke her AFE zone, then the G-spot, and back again. Use clockwise strokes followed by counterclockwise strokes. (Reminder: The AFE zone is a small, sensitive patch of textured skin at the top of the vagina close to the cervix. The G-spot is that spongy mass of rough tissue located on the front wall of the vagina about halfway between the pubic bone and the cervix.) If you're going down on her, don't overlook her U-spot, or the tiny area of tissue above the opening of the urethra (and right below the clitoris). Shift from the C-spot to the U-spot when she is close to orgasm. Tease her by going back and forth until she can't take it anymore.

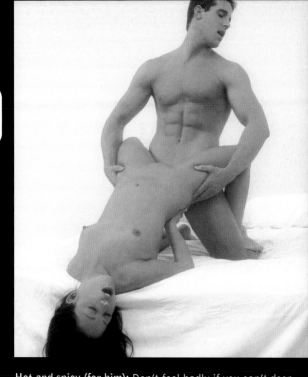

Hot and spicy (for him): Don't feel badly if you can't deep throat his penis without gagging. Concentrate your attention during fellatio on the H-spot (the head of the penis) and the R area (the visible line along the center of the scrotum); alternatively, stroke his P zone (the 1-inch area between the anus and the base of the scrotum). Connect these three dots and chances are he won't notice or care that you don't take the entire shaft into your mouth!

Hot Spot Intercourse

The Sexy Setup

Here's a fun game that combines hitting the hot spots and intercourse—what more could you ask for? Tell your lover you've got a game that's sure to hit all the right spots— and send him over the edge!

Rules & Tools

Be forewarned: Some of these positions may take a little practice, and some require a certain amount of flexibility! Set a sexy scene, dim the lights, and do some light stretches beforehand to get warmed up and build the sexual tension.

Playing the Game

Sweet and safe: In the missionary position, put your feet on his shoulders or pull your knees up to your chest and place your feet flat against his chest. Alternatively, have him hold your legs with his forearms under the knees. If you're on top, either lean back or forward, which is more effective at hitting the hot spots than riding straight up and down. When using the spoon position, lie on your side with your back to him, bent slightly at the knees and waist. He enters you from behind, also bent slightly at the knees and waist.

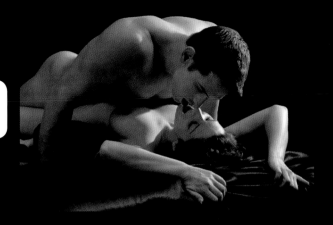

Hot and Spicy: Try the X position, which is adapted from the Kama Sutra position called "Woman acting the part of man." Imagine that your bodies form an X, with the connection at the genitals. He sits at the edge of the bed with his back straight and one leg outstretched on the bed, the other outstretched toward the floor, or, if he prefers, braced up on a straight-backed chair placed by the bed. Support your back with pillows, then sit astride your partner with both legs braced on his shoulders.

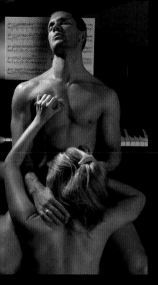

Drawwwww Out His Pleasure

The Sexy Setup

Text your lover and tell him you've got a game to play that's designed especially for him. The goal: to prolong his pleasurable sensations as long as possible without launching the rocket!

Rules & Tools

Set a sexy scene, whether that means making the bed with silk sheets or setting up a love nest in front of a burning fireplace. Dim the lights or light some candles, open a bottle of wine, and stash some lubricant or sex toys nearby for use if desired.

Playing the Game

Sweet and safe: First things first: Heat up your man in whatever way you like best—kiss him all over, manhandle his penis, or perform oral sex—whatever it takes to get

63

him hard and ready. Then practice the Three-Finger Draw, a simple and effective technique that's been used in China for five thousand years. As you're sucking his penis, locate the midpoint of his perineum, or that sensitive area between the base of the testicles and the anus. As soon as you feel like he's going to come, curve the three longest fingers of your right hand very slightly and apply pressure—not too light and not too hard—to this spot. The trick is in finding the right spot and applying the pressure in the nick of time, which may take a little practice. Chances are he won't complain if you need to try, try again!

Hot and Spicy: This technique, called the Big Draw, requires your lover to have a strong PC muscle. Heat him up as only you know best, then outline the technique. When he feels he's just about to come, have him stop thrusting and pull back to approximately 1 inch of penetration (but don't withdraw completely). Have him flex the PC muscle and hold to a count of nine, or flex nine times in rapid succession. (Have him try it both ways!) Resume thrusting with shallow strokes and repeat! Ready to step it up? Have him practice a Taoist technique called Count the Strokes. As he's thrusting, have him count out sets of shallow, then deep, strokes. In the classic "set of nines," he makes nine shallow strokes (without ever withdrawing completely), then one deep one, then eight shallow strokes, then two deep ones, and so forth. If you lose yourself in this game, whose counting, anyway?

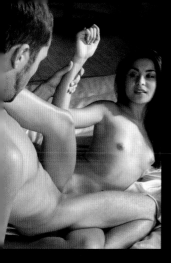

Spike My Oh!

The Sexy Setup

Every man does something special just before he's going to orgasm. The goal of this game? To identify his "moment" and spike his orgasm, otherwise known as triggering it yourself!

Rules & Tools

You've got to do your homework before you can play this game: Pay attention to the subtle signs that your lover is close to coming, whether he holds his breath, breathes more intensely, or makes a certain sound. Once you've studied (and verified!) his particular moment, pull the shades, light some candles, and wear your sexiest lingerie.

Playing the Game

Sweet and safe: Use your favorite moves to get your man fully aroused. When you feel he's ready to come, spike his orgasm, or "trigger" it yourself, by pinching, or biting his nipples right at the moment of orgasm. Another easy but effective maneuver: pause. If he's on top, grab his buttocks at the moment of orgasm. Use your PC muscle to pull him in a little deeper, and make eye contact with him. Ready to step it up? Just as he's about to come, stimulate his G-spot with your thumb or finger pressed gently on his perineum. Alternatively, if he's comfortable, insert a well-lubed finger inside his anus to stimulate the G-spot from inside.

Hot and Spicy: If he's on top and close to orgasm, grab his hip bones or buttocks and rock him, side to side, or back and forth. When you control the direction of his pelvic moments, you also control the speed of thrusting and the depth of penetration. To him, it feels like you are pulling the orgasm out of him in a very explosive way. Alternatively, if you're on top and he's close to orgasm, put your hands on his hips and pull him toward you. Keep your body weight on your knees so you don't bear down on his hips. Want to give him something really special? Fellate him to orgasm. When you feel he's ready to come, take his pelvis in both hands and rock him toward you so that he goes deeper into your mouth. Ready for the ultimate move? Master the Butterfly Quiver. When he's very hard, move so you're on top. Flex your PC muscle in a continuous pattern of tightening (as you pull him inside) and releasing (as you push him out), replicating the pattern of a butterfly's pulsating wings.

Classic 69
(and Then Some!)

The Sexy Setup

This is an easy game to pitch to your lover: You'll both get your share of oral pleasure. What's more, while everyone knows the meaning of 69, you may learn a few new variations on this classic position for oral sex!

Rules & Tools

This game takes a little concentration, as you're going to lick, suck, and use your tongue to give him (or her) a mind-blowing orgasm while he (or she) returns the favor. This may take practice, so don't beat yourself up if you lose yourself in your orgasm and have to pick up the reins and finish his afterward.

Playing the Game

Sweet and safe: Lie side by side with your lover, and rest your head on her inner thigh. (She can rest her head on your inner thigh.) Imagine her genital area as a flower that you are slowly and gently going to open up using your tongue and lips. Gently tease and kiss around her outer labia, using your fingers to part them slightly. Use your tongue to feel for her inner lips, then flick her clitoris once or twice. Insert

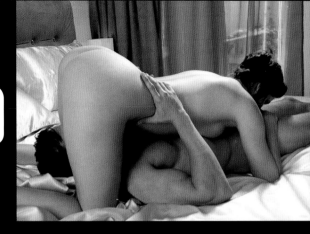

a finger into her vagina or her anus, then slowly increase the intensity and duration of your tongue on her clitoris. Use your fingers to gently expose the clit completely and use gentle laps of your tongue to bring her over the top. As you do this, ask your lover to practice her favorite oral sex techniques on your rock-hard penis.

Hot and Spicy: Try these variations on the classic 69: Have your lover lie on top of you, facing your feet, knees at your shoulders and her genitals in your face. Prop a pillow under your head so you can reach her clitoris without straining your neck! Alternatively, lie on top of her and bury your head between her thighs. Your penis will dangle right over her mouth! Last but not least, try the Curled 69: Curl into a tucked position for a tighter, more intimate version of the classic oral sex thriller.

Queen for a Day

The Sexy Setup

Tell your lover you're her adoring knight, and you want to treat her like a queen. Specifically, you've got a seat of honor that promises hours of pleasure!

Rules & Tools

This is all about pleasuring your lover, so be prepared to spend some time on your knees, exploring all her most glorious treasures. If you want to get into role-playing, dress like a squire or knight, and ask her to dress like a queen. Then set up a throne by draping furs or velvet over a chair and giving her a crown. Bring along a silk tie for blindfolding. If you're not on a bed or other soft surface, put a blanket or pillow under her knees. Explain to her that she's in control—while you're there to pleasure her orally, she can control the intensity by moving up and down on your tongue. If she needs something to hold on to, position yourselves so she can lean her hands against the wall.

Playing the Game

Sweet and safe: Lead your lover to her throne, perhaps blindfolded so she doesn't know what awaits her. Slowly and seductively remove her clothing, or, if you're playing a game

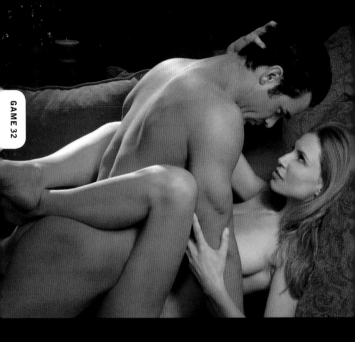

of stolen royal love along the lines of Catherine Howard, the wife of Henry VIII who had an affair with Thomas Culpeper, lift up her skirts and bury your face in her vulva. Start by kissing her inner thighs and taking in the smell and taste of her vulva. Give her genitals long, slow, wet kisses, then introduce your tongue for exploring her labia, crevices, and clitoris. Find a rhythm she likes to give her a mind-blowing orgasm fit for a queen! Alternatively, have your lover kneel above your face so you can use your kisses and tongue to explore her labia and clitoris; run your tongue from her vagina to her anus and back again, all the while gently massing her buttocks. Put a finger or two inside her vagina and play with her G-spot while you bring her to orgasm with your tongue.

Hot and Spicy: In this scenario, pretend you are a foreign knight who has taken the queen hostage. Your duty: not to hurt her, but to pleasure her beyond her wildest dreams. Lead her to her throne, but then tie her hands to the chair. Spread her legs and tie her legs to the chair as well. Now she's your captive, and you can tease her until she screams for mercy—or moans with pleasure! Ready to step it up? Put together a "Royal Tool Kit" full of her favorite sex toys and props, then use them one by one while she's strapped to the chair. Use a finger vibrator to stimulate her nipples while you lick her clitoris, or bring her to orgasm manually while you penetrate her with a dildo. Talk about your majesty's secret service!

Oral Sex Slave

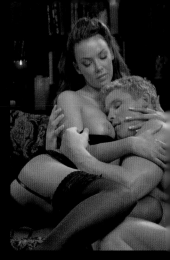

The Sexy Setup

What man doesn't relish the thought of his own personal sex slave? But the twist in this game is that it's all about pleasuring him using oral sex. Ladies, get on your knees and service your master!

Rules & Tools

Set up a pleasure den using soft blankets, furs, or silk sheets. Dress the part as you see fit: Wear your sexiest lingerie and high heels, a maiden's dress with no under-garments, a leather jacket and boots (otherwise naked!), or a collar and nothing else. Bring along soft ties for gentle bondage if desired.

Playing the Game

Sweet and safe: Lead your lover to his pleasure den, and ask him where he most likes to be kissed. Start kissing him there, but then take your kisses to his neck, his chest, his belly, and downward. Kiss him all over, but avoid the genitals and tease him until he orders you to touch him there. Then suck, nibble, and bite your way around until he orders you to make him come. Alternatively, lie down and have him kneel in front of you so his penis is right in front of your mouth (you may need a pillow or two to get the angle right). Hold his penis with one hand and explore his backside with the other; fondle his testicles, insert a finger in his anus, or just lightly trace your fingertips along his perineum as you suck him off.

Hot and Spicy: Before you begin the actual sex play, ask him what he'd like to eat and drink, then sit on his lap and hand feed him grapes or let him sip champagne. Shower him with affection while he relaxes and unwinds, but then surprise him suddenly by tying him to the chair (a short struggle will turn you both on!) and removing just enough of his clothes to reveal his genitals. Although he's the master, he's also your prisoner, and you intend to draw out your pleasurable torture. Undress seductively and tease him in a sexy manner, all the while knowing he cannot touch you. When he's sufficiently turned on, get on your knees and suck him off as you know best.

8 Days a Week

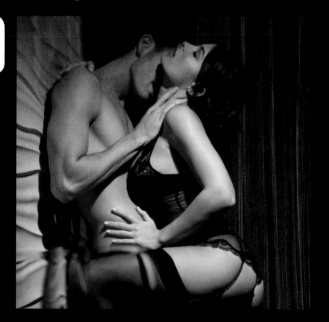

The Sexy Setup

Remember the Beatles song, "8 Days a Week"? This extended game is all about drawing out the pleasure— and teasing your lover over several days—in order to give him the orgasm of his life.

Rules & Tools

This game doesn't have to be played over 7 days. It could take place over a weekend, with the pleasure given every few hours—or you can really make the work week hum by by giving a small amount of pleasure every night, but holding off on letting him come until the last night. The rules are simple: Use your oral sex techniques every day (or every few hours) to stimulate him, but don't let him come until you're ready. It will be a challenge for you to pull away, but even harder for him to know he's got to wait for his orgasm!

Playing the Game

Sweet and safe: Sing to the tune of the Beatles song, but use these naughty lyrics instead:

Ooh I need your cock, babe,
Guess you know it's true.
Hope you need my lips, babe,
Just like I need you.
Hold me, kiss me, hold me, suck you.
I ain't got nothin' but blow jobs,
Eight days a week.

Day #1: Wet your lips and run your tongue around the head of his penis to moisten it. Hold the base of his penis firmly in one hand, then form the ring and the seal with your other hand. Use that hand in a twisting motion as you fellate him. Get him stimulated, but stop well before orgasm.

Day #2: Circle the head of his penis with your tongue in a swirling motion, and then work your tongue in long strokes up and down his shaft. Again, get him stimulated but don't let him come.

Day #3: Follow the ridge of the corona with your tongue while working the shaft with your hands, the penis sandwiched between them.

Day #4: Strum the frenulum with your tongue and lick the raphe. Make eye contact with him from time to time.

Day #5: Repeatedly pull his penis into your mouth, then push it out, using suction while keeping the tongue in motion.

Day #6: Go back to the head. Swirl your tongue around it. Suck the head. Swirl. Suck. Repeat. Repeat.

Day #7: Use one or all of the above techniques to get him off!

Hot and Spicy: Use the timeline and techniques already listed, but step it up by introducing gentle bondage, an anal butt plug, or gentle nipple clamps. Ready for even racier sex play? Bring a friend along, blindfold your lover, and take turns stimulating him. Remember, don't let him come until the final day!

Stranger Danger

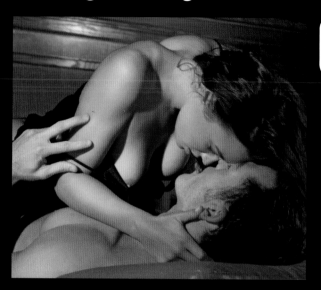

The Sexy Setup

This is a great game to play with a longtime lover, as it brings out the "danger" and "secret" elements of having sex with a stranger or in a public place. Tell your lover you're going to play a game where he's the pickup target, but you're calling the shots.

Rules & Tools

Make a plan ahead of time with your lover, then send him a sexy note to remind him of the details. "Meet me at Oliver's at 8 pm; be sure to bring a hard-on."

Playing the Game

Sweet and safe: Dress as if you're out to pick up a man: Try a new top with a plunging neckline or short skirt. Instruct your lover to find a spot at the bar, order a drink, and relax. Then do your best to flirt him up: Play hard to get, act like a tease, or flirt openly. Draw out the pickup as long as possible, then lead him to your car and continue teasing him by licking and sucking his penis. If you want to draw out the pleasure, leave him panting for more but go back to the bar. Pick up where you left off once you get home!

Hot and Spicy: Play the part of a slut or prostitute. Tease him with your eyes or hands, brush up against him suggestively, or touch his package when no one's looking. Whisper what you'd like to do to him while you lean over and expose your cleavage. Alternatively, invite a female friend to join in (but don't tell your lover). Ask your friend to flirt with your man openly—a little competition can add some spice to the situation. Have a secret word for when it's time for her to head home. Once he's hot and hard, take him by the hand and give him a steamy blow job in the men's bathroom or a hidden closet—the fear of getting caught will only intensify his orgasm!

Dress for Quickie Success

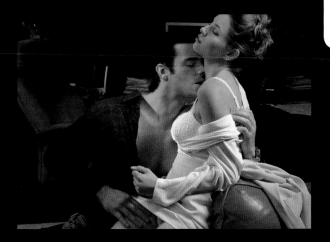

The Sexy Setup

Here's a sexy "dress-up" game that's sure to get you both aroused—and give you ideas for how to dress for quickie success in the future!

Rules & Tools

Anything goes in this game, although the end goal is to walk away with several outfits or costumes that are perfect for quickie sex. Think of this as a road test for all your sexiest clothing that can be pushed aside, unzipped quickly, or just torn off! If you want, make a scorecard and rating system for your lover so he can rank your outfits. Remember, any score is a good score!

Playing the Game

Sweet and safe: Set up a sexy "viewing" area for your lover, whether that's on your bed, in a relaxing chair, or lying naked on a rug! Dim the lights and fix him a cocktail, then ask him to play voyeur for a bit while you model some quickie outfits. Head into your closet and model a variety of push-aside costumes: Try a short skirt with no underwear, a zip-down sweater with no bra underneath, lingerie that can be easily pushed aside, and so on. Be sure to include one outfit that can be ripped off, such as an old t-shirt and a pair of his worn-out boxers. Have your lover rank each outfit for how much it turns him on and how easily he thinks it will work for quickie sex. Feeling randy? Move on to the hot and spicy version of this game.

Hot and Spicy: Set up a timer and see how long it takes your lover to get to down to business, whether that means manhandling your breasts, fondling your buttocks, or exploring your clitoris with his tongue or fingers. If you're feeling especially sexy, try to fight him off—gentle horse-play can add to the excitement. And don't forget the outfit that can be ripped off—a little roughhousing can really heat up the action! Alternatively, set the timer and see how long it takes to reach orgasm using each different outfit.

Quickie Chinese Menu

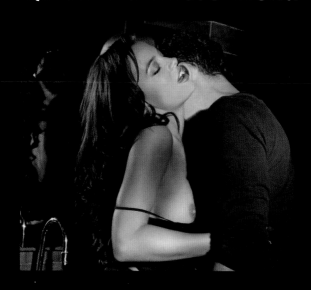

The Sexy Setup

You know the concept of a Chinese food menu—pick one dish from column A, another from column B, and so on until you've built your meal. This game works on the same premise, but you're picking what kind of quickie sex you want and where to have it. Tell your lover you've got a sexy menu of options that need testing, and he's an essential ingredient!

Rules & Tools

Set up a matrix together: Design a grid where column A represents all the different types of quickie sex and column B represents all the assorted places to have that sex. Use your imagination—pick a variety of places in your home, at your office, outdoors, or even in public places such as a furniture store or movie theater.

Playing the Game

Sweet and safe: Close your eyes and put your finger on one of the boxes in the matrix for a quickie surprise. Alternatively, work through the matrix together until there's a check in every box. Options include: Pretend you are meeting your lover in an empty conference room and time is of the essence. Do it in the backyard at midnight, in the restroom of your favorite pub, or in your mother's gazebo.

Hot and Spicy: Add some of these locations to your matrix, then test them out one by one! Have mutual oral sex in the backseat of the car parked in the garage, while the kids are watching a video inside the house. Have sex in a standing position in your bedroom closet while your dinner guests are cleaning up the dishes. Visit your lover at his office and sit on his lap in a desk chair. Sit on top of the running dryer and have your man perform oral sex—the heat and vibrations of the dryer will add to the pleasure! Shopping at the mall? Suck off your man in the men's dressing room, or find a hidden room in a cavernous furniture store.

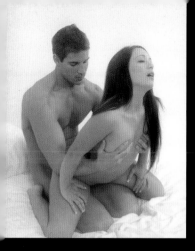

Anal Play 101

The Sexy Setup

If you've never experi-
mented with anal sex
play, here's the game
for you. Tell your lover
you're interested in
exploring her back end,
but promise to take it
slow, talk it through, and change gears if anything feels
awkward or uncomfortable. Then get ready to think about
all things anal, all the time!

Rules & Tools

Set a sexy scene for your backdoor experimentation, and
serve your lover a glass of wine or champagne if she's at
all nervous about this idea. Bring along plenty of lubricant,
use safe practices, and stash your favorite props (feathers
or silk ties) and toys (butt plug, anal beads, or other toys)
nearby if you sense she's at all comfortable with taking
things a little further.

Playing the Game

Sweet and safe: Kiss her deeply and slowly undress her, taking time to caress her neck, arms, and breasts. Tell her how beautiful she is and how excited you are to experiment together. If she's tense, consider bringing her to orgasm before you explore her backside, so she'll be more relaxed. Have her lie on her side or stomach, then gently massage her buttocks. Gently run a finger, feather, or a silk tie very lightly down her crack, then separate her buttocks as you go. Repeat this as necessary, making sure she's aroused before you move to the next step. Tease her buttocks apart using very light strokes, then circle closer to her anus, all the while kissing her lower back or the back of her neck. Apply lubrication to your finger and slowly tease the anal opening, then retreat. Tease and retreat until you're sure she's aroused, then gently insert your finger into her anus and circle inside the opening. Push and pull your finger in and out as if you were having sex; if she's interested, insert a second finger and continue the movement.

Hot and Spicy: Try stimulating her clitoris with your other hand as you move your finger in and out of her anus. Alternatively, masturbate as you touch her anal area, then come onto her lower back. Ready for more advanced techniques? Use a set of anal beads on your lover: Lubricate the beads, insert them gently into her anus, then pull them out, one bead at a time, while you kiss her breasts or lick her clitoris. Use an anal plug while you have sex—your lover may find the double penetration expands her orgasm.

Beyond Doggie-Style

The Sexy Setup

If you've already had anal intercourse and you're ready for experimentation, this position game is just for you. Tell your lover you've got some new ideas for backdoor pleasure that are sure to get him off!

Rules & Tools

Have plenty of lubrication and be sure to use safe practices. Bring along your favorite vibrator if desired. Then let your imagination—or your flexibility—influence the direction of this game.

Playing the Game

Sweet and safe: If you're a beginner when it comes to anal sex, the doggie-style position is easiest. But if you're ready for some variation on that game, lie on your back with your legs straight up or your ankles resting on his shoulders. Have him kneel between your legs, lube things up, and thrust away! Alternatively, have him lie on his back, then lower yourself onto him, either facing him or facing away, or have him sit in a chair or on the bed, then lower yourself onto him, facing away. And the ultimate position for easy anal sex? Spoon style: Lie side by side, with your buttocks against his penis.

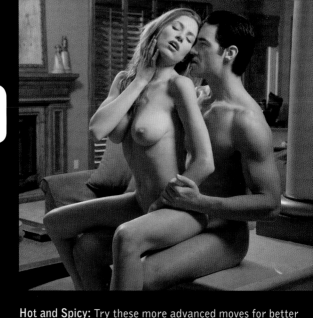

Hot and Spicy: Try these more advanced moves for better anal sex. Stand together in a doorway, with you facing away from your lover. Let him penetrate you as you hold onto the doorframes for leverage! Lean over if you want it hard and deep. Alternatively, have him lie flat on his back, then lower yourself onto him but extend your body so you end up laying flat on top of him, your back to his chest. Ask him to kiss your neck and play with your clitoris as you have anal sex. Last but not least, have him sit on a chair, then lower yourself onto him. Bring along your vibrator and masturbate to clitoral orgasm while he enters your backdoor.

Backdoor Woman

The Sexy Setup

You've heard the phrase backdoor man? This time the roles are reversed: You get to control the action at your male lover's back door. Write your male lover a sexy note and tell him you want to explore his back door. Promise you'll be gentle as you investigate his assets, but you're sure there are some new pleasures zones worth exploring!

Rules & Tools

Line up a number of anal toys for this game and bring along plenty of lubrication. Have these (or other toys) on hand: butt plug, strap-on dildo, anal vibrator, anal beads, or any pocketsize or finger vibrator. Set up a low-lit, sexy scene for this game: Line a couch with fur, create a nest of soft blankets on the floor, or make your bed with silk sheets.

Playing the Game

Sweet and safe: If this is your lover's first time with anal play, take it slow. Dress in your sexiest lingerie and help him loosen up by serving him a drink. Then take out one of your toys and let him look at it close-up. Explain why you think it might turn him on, but be open if he's not interested and simply move on to the next toy. Kiss and caress him in your

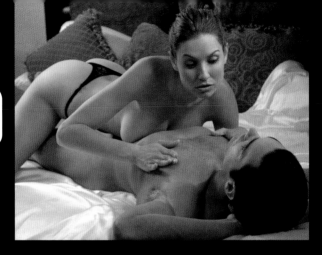

usual way, then slowly move to fondling and sucking his penis and nibbling his testicles. Try running a finger vibrator along his inner thighs, up to his testicles, and along his perineum. Be sure to ask if he likes the feeling, and if he does, continue with your back door play, perhaps inserting the butt plug or anal beads while you suck him off.

Hot and Spicy: You know your man's open to any anal suggestion, so take it up a notch and explore your own fantasies. Lube up the strap on and give it to him up the ass like the strong and sexy backdoor woman you are, or just insert a vibrating butt plug and ride him like a cowgirl! Ready to step it up? Play a game of backdoor woman meets backdoor man. Both of you should chose your favorite butt plug, then have intercourse doggie style!

Position Tic-Tac-Toe

The Sexy Setup

Remember playing tic-tac-toe as a child? This naughty version of the same game can be played over and over—orgasms guaranteed! Write your lover a note and tell him you've got a game to play that will test his ability to have multiple orgasms in multiple positions, and there's a bonus prize to boot.

Rules & Tools

You'll need a simple tic-tac-toe game, which you can purchase beforehand or even just draw on a piece of paper. Make a grid using four lines to create nine different boxes. Set a sexy scene and allow for plenty of time for sex play. Alternatively, use the tic-tac-toe game over a span of days, then reward the winner on the weekend!

Playing the Game

Sweet and safe: Try out each of the six basic positions with the goal of having an orgasm in each position. If he orgasms, he gets to mark an X in one of the tic-tac-toe boxes. If you also orgasm you get to mark an 0 in one of the boxes. Continue testing the positions and marking the boxes until someone wins the game of tic-tac-toe, then determine a bonus prize for the winner, such as a prolonged back

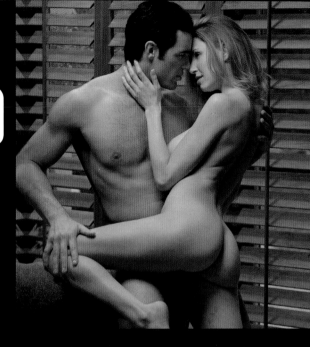

massage, dinner in bed (with both of you naked!), or his choice of the next game to play.

Hot and Spicy: Play tic-tac-toe, but use the grid to mark an X or 0 each time your lover tries a new technique, is willing to experiment with a new move, or plays with a new sex toy. Play for the winner of three out of five or four out of seven games, then reward the winner with his or her choice of role-play games.

Bag of Tricks

The Sexy Setup

You know that most women don't come via sexual intercourse alone, so tell your lover you've got a bag of tricks you'd like to open up to guarantee you come every time you make love!

Rules & Tools

Bring along your favorite assorted tools for stimulating your clitoris, whether that's your hand, a finger vibe, or his penis. Set a sexy scene, such as a soft rug in front of the fireplace, a pleasure den on your living room floor, or a nest of blankets in your bed.

Playing the Game

Sweet and safe: Kiss, fondle, and caress your lover as you know best, then get naked together using slow and sensual movements. Once you're ready for intercourse, have him enter you manually, then try this simple move for stimulating your clitoris when the space between you is tight. Insert two fingers of one hand between your bodies and form an upside-down V shape with your fingers straddling your clitoris.

Press the V in time with his thrusting. Alternatively, if he's entered you spoon-style from behind, take his fingers and

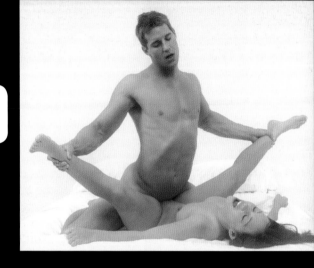

place them in the V shape on the sides of your clitoris. Grind against his fingers as he thrusts from behind.

Hot and Spicy: Ready to try some other moves? Kneel together on the bed and have him enter you from behind. Place one hand on the bed frame and use the other hand to masturbate while he thrusts from behind. Have him lie flat on his back, then lower yourself onto him. Once you're in position, lean backward, resting on one hand. Use the other hand to stimulate your clitoris using a finger vibe. Lie on your side, with him on his side between your legs. Wrap your legs around his back. As you control the thrusting movement, have him insert a well-lubed finger between you so he can tickle your clitoris.

The Bucking Cowgirl Meets the Missionary Man

The Sexy Setup

You know the female and male superior positions by heart: cowgirl and missionary man. Tell your lover you've got a game that's sure to increase the odds of reaching orgasm in either position!

Rules & Tools

Set a sexy scene, such as a soft rug in front of the fireplace, a pleasure den on your living room floor, or a nest of blankets in your bed, and bring along your favorite sex toys if desired. Then let your imagination take over!

Playing the Game

Sweet and safe: Here's how to make the cowgirl an even better orgasm position: Alternate deep thrusting with using the head of his penis to stimulate your clitoris. Move from side to side rather than up and down. When orgasm is imminent, flatten yourself out on top of him, clench your thighs together, and grind your clitoris into him as you flex

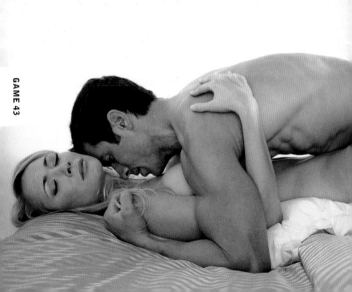

slightly forward as you push down on his penis, stimulating your clitoris. Pull up and move slightly backward on the upstroke, stimulating your G-spot. Use your hand if you need to and don't forget to flex your PC muscle.

Hot and Spicy: Make the missionary position even better with this set of tricks: Place a pillow(s) beneath the small of your back to change the angle of penetration to one of greater depth. Lie on your back with your legs up as straight and high as they will comfortably go. He kneels in front of you. This tightens your vagina, providing greater friction for both of you, and it leaves your hands free to play with your clitoris. Lie on your back and put your legs over his shoulders. Lift one leg up and put it over his shoulder or around his back. Put your feet on his chest or shoulders and bend your knees inward, again to change the angle of penetration and control the thrust. Wrap your legs around his waist or his neck for the same reasons. Have him pull you to the edge of the bed and hold your legs as he enters you from a standing position.

Spoonful of Loving Meets the Backdoor Man

The Sexy Setup

You know the spooning and backdoor positions by heart. Tell your lover you've got a game that's sure to increase the odds of reaching orgasm in either position!

Rules & Tools

Set a sexy scene, such as a pleasure den of soft blankets, furs, and pillows on your living room floor. Dim the lights or light some candles and bring along your favorite sex toys if desired.

Playing the Game

Sweet and safe: Here's how to make side by side, also known as spooning, a better orgasm position: Either you or he should stimulate your clitoris. Start by adding a vibrator—this is a great position for vibe play because your hands are free. Make this your go-to position when he's tired, but you want sex. Masturbate first until you are highly aroused, then let him enter you from behind. Touch yourself while he thrusts away, and try to time your orgasm to his!

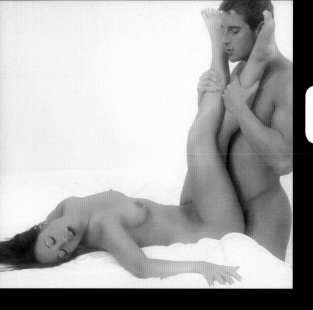

Hot and Spicy: Ready to freshen up that old doggie-style position? Try these moves for better orgasms: Lower your upper body so that your chest touches the bed. This elongates your vaginal barrel, making a tighter fit for his penis. If he typically grabs your hips or ass and controls the thrusting, ask him to caress your vulva and finger your clitoris while otherwise remaining relatively still. Then you thrust back against him. Alternatively, try the rear-entry position lying down, with you on your stomach. Clench your thighs together after he enters you and lift one leg for deeper penetration.

Sitting Lotus Meets the Stand-up Man

The Sexy Setup

You know the sitting and standing positions by heart. Tell your lover you've got a game that's sure to increase the odds of reaching orgasm in either position!

Rules & Tools

Establish an erotic mood with candles, wine, sexy clothing, or music—whatever turns you on and gets you tingly all over. Bring along your favorite sex toys or silk ties for gentle bondage if desired.

Playing the Game

Sweet and safe: Here's how to make the sitting position even hotter: Have your lover grasp your buttocks firmly, then lean backward as he thrusts. Add a vibrator, especially a vibrating cock ring on him or a strap-on vibe for you.

Hot and Spicy: Use these moves to bring your standing position to new heights of passion! Change the depth and angle of penetration by doing it on the stairs, with you one

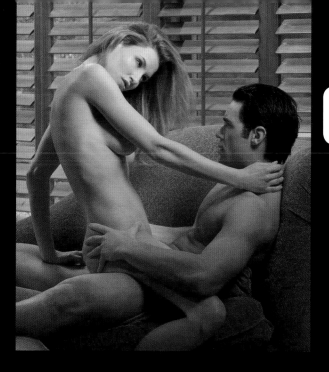

step above him. Alternatively, stand in front of him, facing in the opposite direction, and bend slightly forward. You'll feel more G-spot stimulation this way. Last but not least, sit on the kitchen counter, washer or dryer, or a high bar stool—whatever is the right height for him to enter you.

Expanding His and Her Orgasms

The Sexy Setup

If you love the idea of orgasm, then chances are you'll relish the idea of expanding an orgasm so it becomes a full-body or even body-mind-spirit experience. Write your lover a romantic note and tell him you've got a game that will spread your orgasm beyond the usual boundaries and stretch his orgasm into new territories!

Rules & Tools

You can use these masturbation techniques alone beforehand for practice, but they can also be used with your lover for communicating how you want to be touched. Set a sexy scene for your love play, such as a nest of blankets in your bed or a soft rug set in front of a roaring fire. Bring along extra pillows for good positioning and viewing and your favorite sex toys if desired.

Playing the Game

Sweet and Safe (for her): Using your fingers or a vibrator, masturbate in a comfortable position. As soon as you become highly aroused, use one hand to massage the area of your vulva, inner thighs, and groin with light, shallow

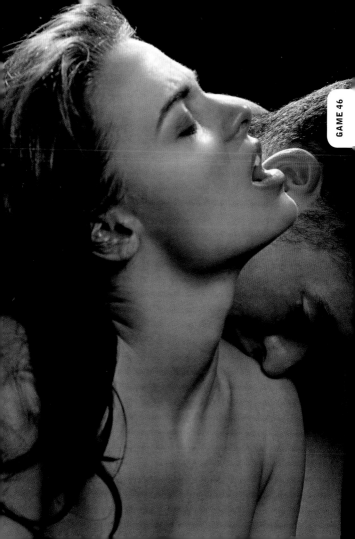

strokes. Imagine that you are spreading your arousal throughout those areas. Continue the massage throughout your orgasm, imagining you are spreading your orgasm into your body. After orgasm, continue rhythmic stroking of your genital area. Feel the orgasm continuing to spread throughout your body for several seconds after it normally would have dissipated.

Sweet and safe (for him): Have your lover masturbate without ejaculating as long as he can. Ten to fifteen minutes is a reasonable goal, though this may not be possible not the first time. Have him do this by stopping or changing strokes when ejaculation is imminent. Have him count the contractions he feels upon ejaculation, normally between three and eight. Note the level and order of intensity. Typically the strongest contractions will be at the beginning. The next time he masturbates, again delay ejaculation as long as possible. This time when he comes, have him flex his PC muscle as if he's trying to stop ejaculation. Then have him continue stimulating his penis very slowly—or do it for him—while squeezing throughout the ejaculation, thus pushing the sensations on and on.

Expanding Orgasms Together

The Sexy Setup

If you've mastered the technique of expanding your orgasm through masturbation, you're ready to step it up and expand your orgasms together.

Rules & Tools

Take a cool, not hot, shower together. Your skin should be cool to each other's touch as you begin.

Playing the Game

Sweet and safe: Lie on the bed side by side, facing one another, with your legs entwined in a scissors position. Insert his flaccid penis into your vagina. Remain still. If necessary, put your hand around the base of his penis to keep it inside until he has a moderate erection. (But don't work to make him have one!) Breathing deeply, try to remain motionless for fifteen minutes. During this time, caress each other's faces, necks, and upper bodies, and make frequent, prolonged eye contact. Whisper terms of endearment. Are you feeling a sense of erotic peace? Now begin moving together. He should be thrusting slowly and gently and you should match his pace with your pelvis and

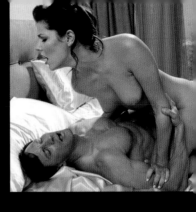

hips. Kiss deeply. As you move your bodies, use your hands to stroke each other, working upward from one another's genitals. Imagine that you are spreading fire with your hands. Resist the desire to move faster when you reach that agonizing point of being "almost there." You want to stay on the verge for as long as possible—until you realize that you are having an orgasm that seems to last forever.

Hot and Spicy: Repeat the sweet and safe game, but try to remain motionless for thrity minutes. As you begin moving together, make your thrusting motions slow and prolonged. Kiss deeply with your eyes open, and try to maintain eye contact as you begin caressing and stroking each other. Whisper how your hands are spreading fire from his penis upward, or as his hands glide from your genitals to your buttocks, nipples, belly, and back again. Hold on to the drawn-out pace as long as possible—your goal is to reach the edge and stay there as long as possible before you both orgasm. Try to maintain eye contact the entire time for the ultimate intimate connection.

Karezza

The Sexy Setup

An Italian word that means "caress," Karezza was developed by an American physician in 1883. As a technique for prolonging intercourse, Karezza is simple and effective and can be practiced in any position. It also encourages extended orgasm—and what woman doesn't like the promise of that reward?

Rules & Tools

Any intercourse position can work for Karezza, but man on top or missionary is least likely to work, so woman on top or side by side are better choices.

Playing the Game

Sweet and safe: The key is to dramatically limit your genital movement. You do not move inside your lover unless you become flaccid. Then you take only shallow strokes to revive your erection. Your lover is allowed to move, including thrusting her hips against yours and contracting her PC muscle around your penis. No matter how excited she gets,

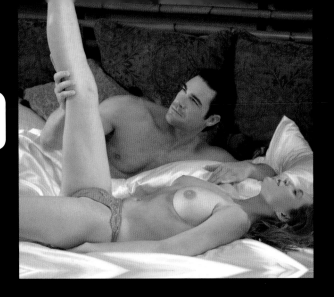

you should only take sufficient thrusting strokes to maintain an erection. Using the masturbation technique of expanding or "spreading," she can encourage the spread of her orgasm throughout her body.

Hot and Spicy: Hold the lovemaking embrace until she has had several orgasms, then move with more energy and satisfy yourself!

Kabbazah

The Sexy Setup

Kabbazah was developed thousands of years ago in the Middle East. A woman who had mastered the French art of pompoir (control of the PC muscle) was called a kabbazah, or "one who holds." Kabbazahs were the best prostitutes in many Eastern countries, including China, Japan, and India. This game won't be a hard sell to your lover: Just tell him you've learned an ancient trick practiced by prostitutes that's guaranteed to intensify his pleasure!

Rules & Tools

There are two absolute requirements for Kabbazah: He must be in a relaxed and receptive state of mind and body. His passivity is crucial. This is not the kind of sex you have when you are desperately tearing each other's clothing off. Second, you must have a virtuoso vagina. Don't even try this until you have diligently practiced Kegels for a period of three weeks to a month.

Playing the Game

Sweet and safe: Begin in the female superior or sitting intercourse position. You should stimulate your lover until he is just erect, not highly aroused. Then insert his penis, but instruct him not to move his pelvis at all. You

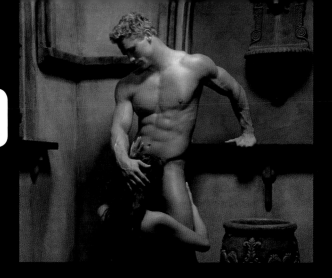

should also strive for no pelvic movement, confining all movements—or as much as possible—to your PC muscle. You may, however, caress and kiss each other. Flex your PC muscle in varying patterns until you feel his penis throbbing, which should occur approximately fifteen minutes into Kabbazah. At that point, he should be highly aroused—so let him take over and orgasm.

Hot and Spicy: Play the sweet and safe version of the game, but when you feel his penis throbbing don't hand over the controls. Instead, time your contractions to the throbbing of his penis, clenching and releasing in time with him. In another ten to fifteen minutes, he may experience a longer, more intense orgasm than ever before.

The Whole Body Orgasm

The Sexy Setup

The whole body orgasm is the result of intense connections on three levels: emotional, sensual, and sexual. Tell your lover that in order to reach this state you'll need to jourey through three doors together.

Rules & Tools

The kiss is particularly intimate and sacred in Tantra, and the belief is that during the kiss, the soul and energy of one partner flows into the other, and vice versa. To experience a whole body orgasm you'll need to master the Tantric yoga kiss, the Yabyum.

Playing the Game

Sweet and safe: During intercourse (in any position), have him practice delaying his orgasm and ejaculation. When you feel your own orgasm is imminent, signal him to stop moving. Then sit in the middle of the bed with his penis inside you, legs wrapped around each other, moving as little as possible. Pressing your foreheads together, breathe into each other's mouths. As he exhales, you inhale, and vice versa. Prolong this "kiss" until remaining still is no longer an option.

Movement will trigger orgasm. The long, slow arousal period and the emotional intensity of the kiss can combine to make your orgasm feel like a whole body experience.

Hot and Spicy: The Yabyum, a Tantric version of the Western sitting position, is a must-try for experiencing whole body orgasm. It is highly touted by sexologists as the ultimate position for prolonging male arousal and intensifying lovers' intimate connection. Sit in the center of the bed facing each other. Wrap your legs around one another so you are sitting on his thighs. Place your right hands at the back of each other's neck, your left hands on each other's tailbones. Now stroke each other's back, using upward strokes only. Look deeply into one another's eyes as you kiss with eyes open. Put his semi-erect penis inside your vagina so it exerts as much indirect pressure as possible on your clitoris and makes G-spot contact. (You can sit on pillows rather than his thighs, if necessary, to get the angle of penetration right.) Perform the Tantric kiss described earlier. Rock slowly together while continuing to rub each other's back and sustaining deep eye contact. Maintain this position until you both orgasm.

Alternatively, try the Passion Flower: As in the Yabyum, start in the center of the bed, facing one another. Wrap your legs comfortably around his body. You can either sit on his thighs or on pillows positioned in front of him. Splay your legs out straight or bend them at the knees, whichever is more comfortable for him. Place your right hands on each other's neck and your left hands at the base of

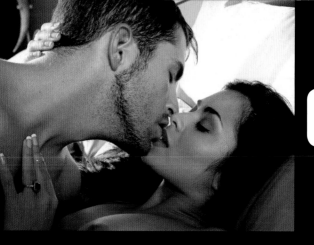

each other's spine. Stroke each other's back, using upward strokes only. Look into each other's eyes and kiss with eyes open. Continue kissing and stroking until you're both highly aroused. Insert his erect penis into your vagina so that the shaft exerts as much indirect pressure on your clitoris as possible. Rock together, slowly rubbing each other's backs and kissing deeply. You may reach orgasm quickly in this position. After your first orgasm (or sooner, if you don't feel orgasm is imminent) try this variation: Have him sit on the bed with his legs open wide. You should lie back on the bed, facing him, with your body between his legs. He lifts your ankles up against his shoulders and enters you at a comfortable angle. Keep your thighs closed, creating a tighter grip on his penis and use one hand to stimulate your clitoris.